PILATES

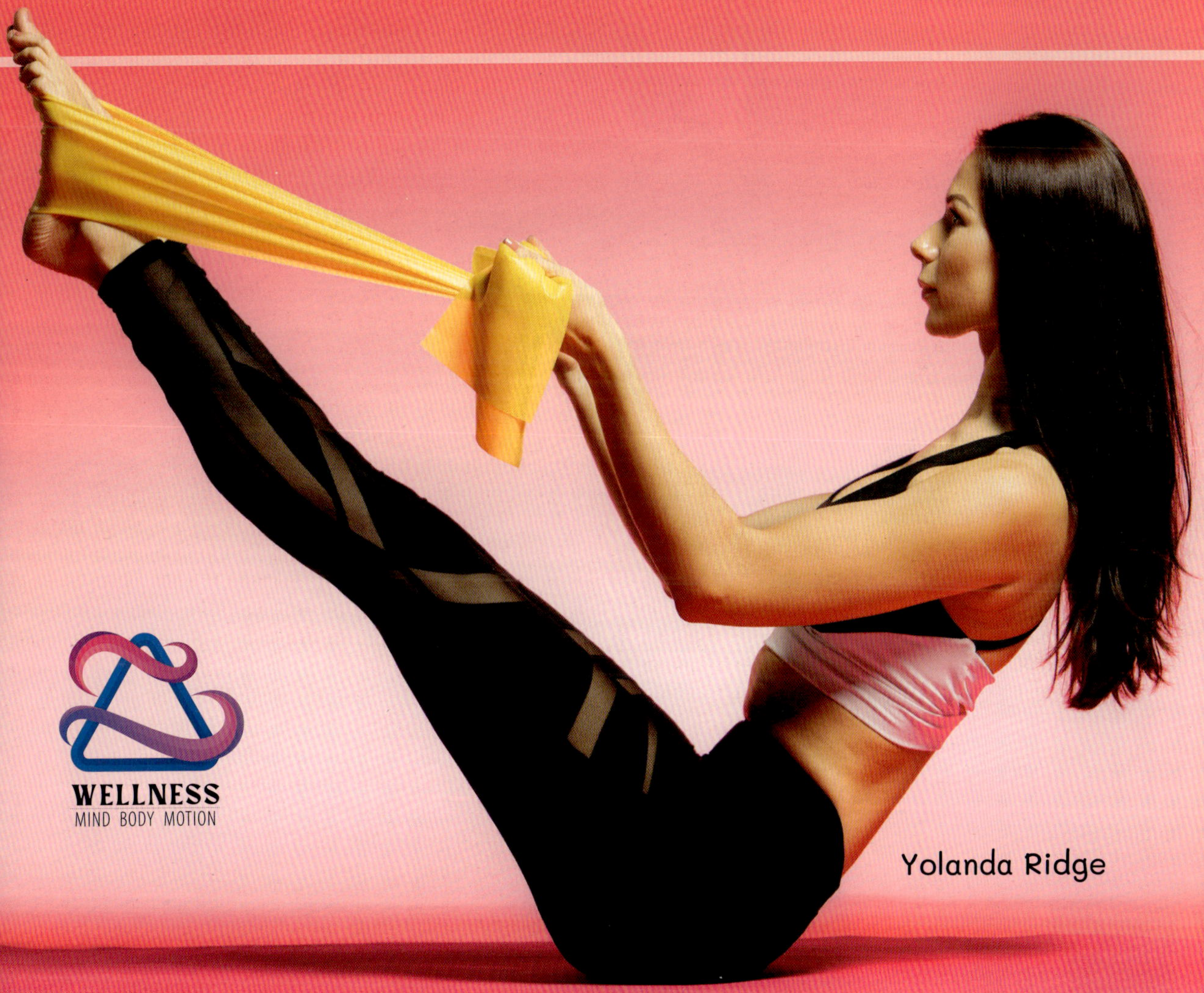

WELLNESS
MIND BODY MOTION

Yolanda Ridge

AV2
www.openlightbox.com

AV2

Step 1
Go to **www.openlightbox.com**

Step 2
Enter this unique code
YVLBUSLW1

Step 3
Explore your interactive eBook!

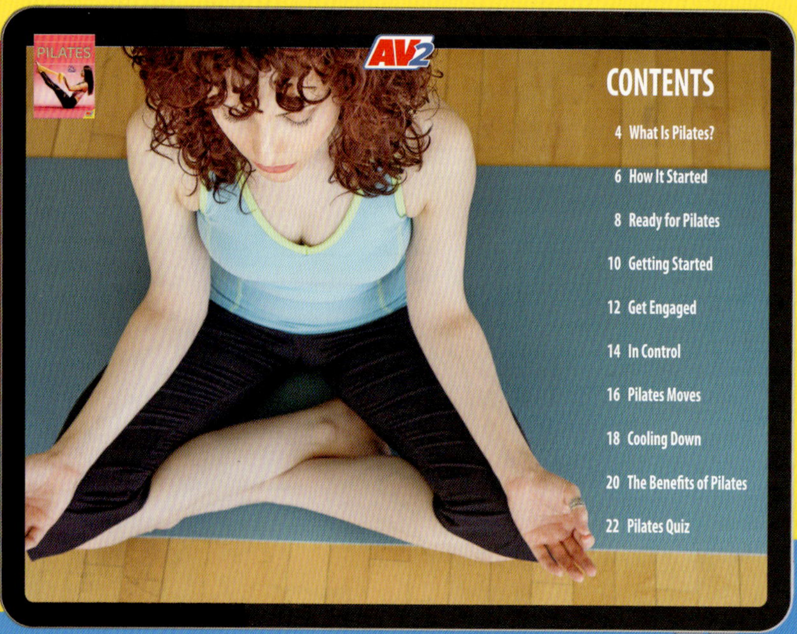

AV2 is optimized for use on any device

Your interactive eBook comes with...

Contents
Browse a live contents page to easily navigate through resources

Audio
Listen to sections of the book read aloud

Videos
Watch informative video clips

Weblinks
Gain additional information for research

Slideshows
View images and captions

Try This!
Complete activities and hands-on experiments

Key Words
Study vocabulary, and complete a matching word activity

Quizzes
Test your knowledge

Share
Share titles within your Learning Management System (LMS) or Library Circulation System

Citation
Create bibliographical references following the Chicago Manual of Style

This title is part of our AV2 digital subscription

1-Year 3–8 Subscription
ISBN 978-1-7911-3306-1

Access hundreds of AV2 titles with our digital subscription.
Sign up for a FREE trial at **www.openlightbox.com/trial**

WELLNESS
MIND BODY MOTION

PILATES

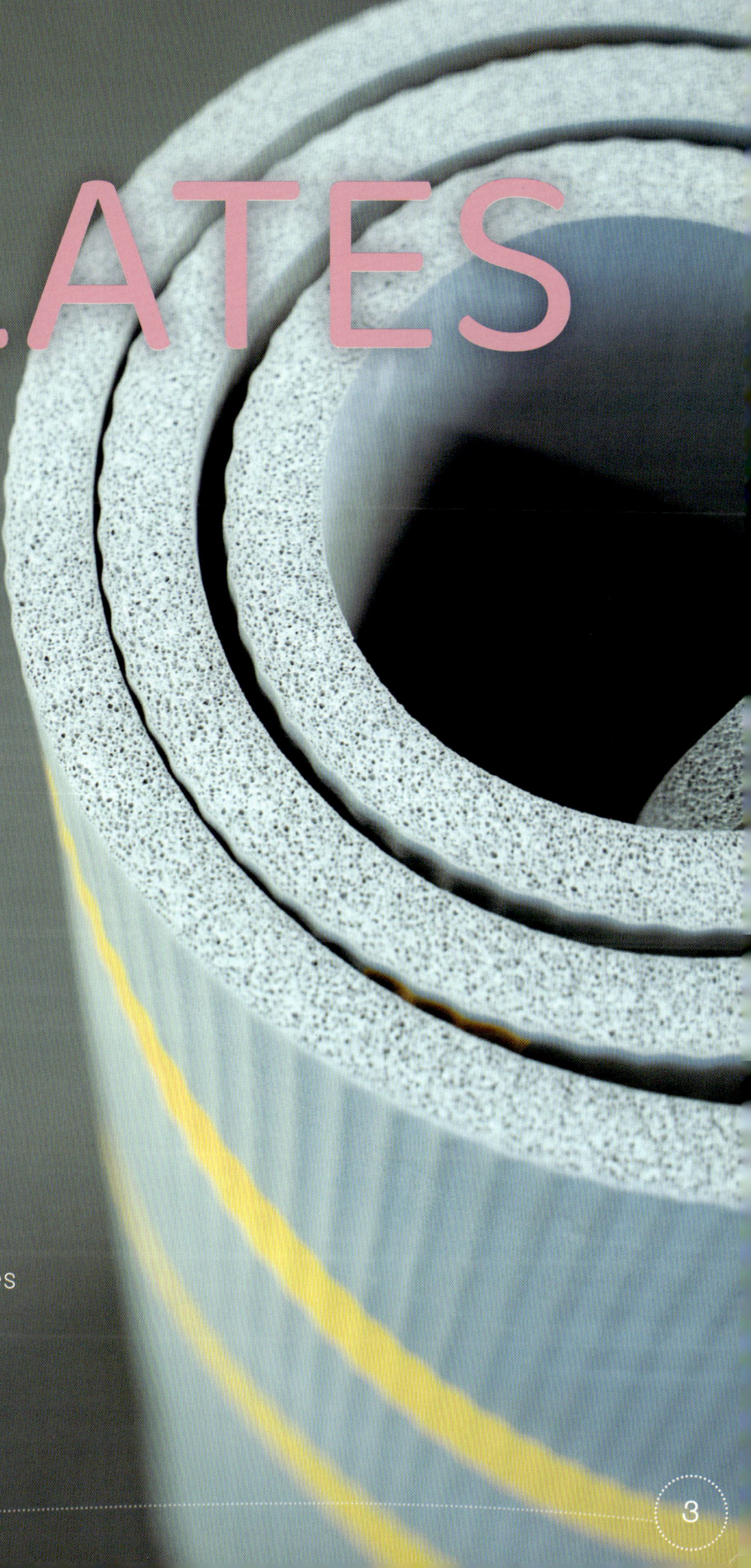

What Is Pilates?

Pilates is a popular form of exercise for people who want to get strong and toned. It helps to strengthen the body's muscles. Pilates uses movements that focus on the **core muscles**. Strong core muscles can help a person develop better **posture**, balance, and **flexibility**.

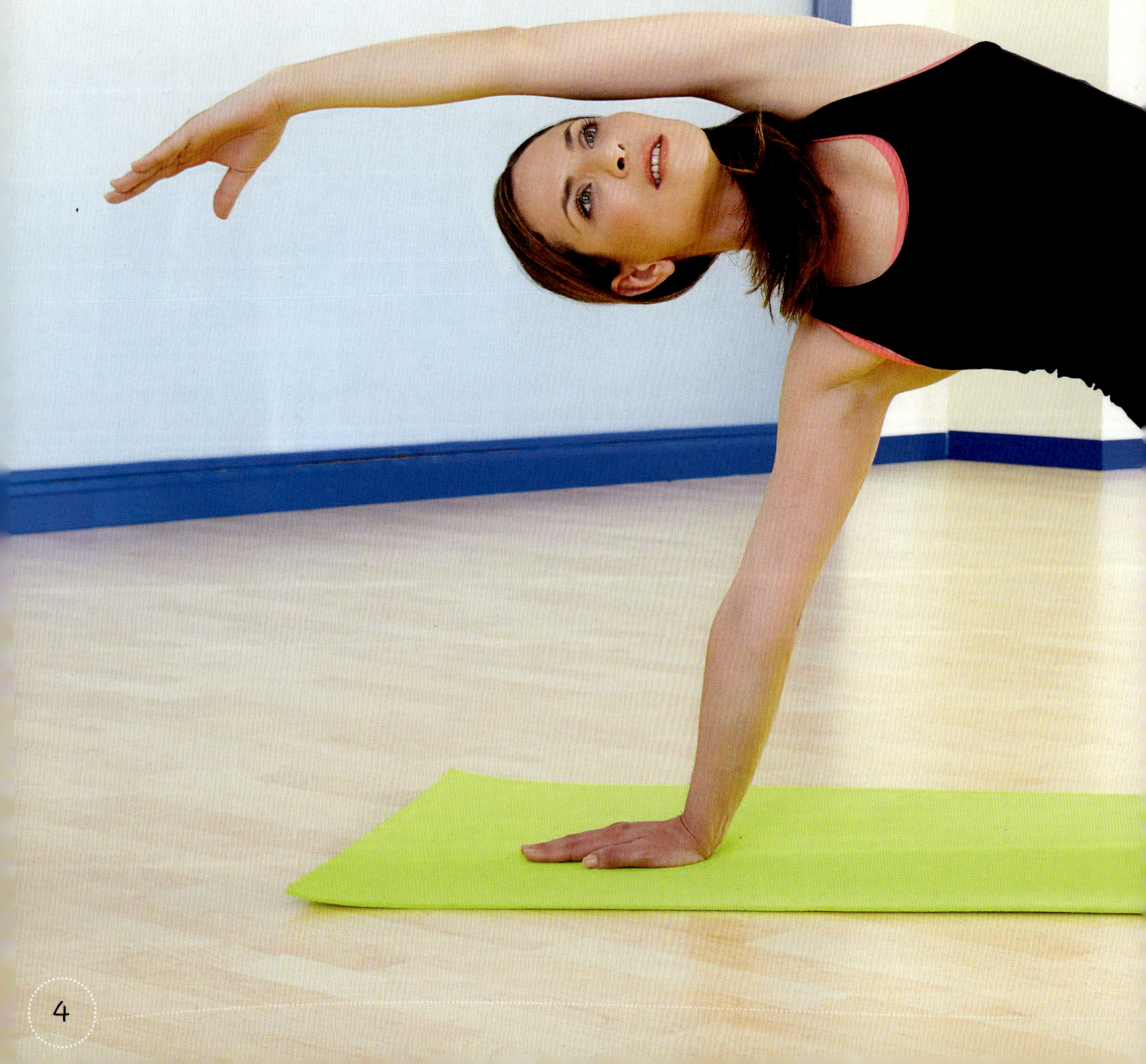

Some Pilates exercises look simple. However, they all require **precision** and control. The mind-body connection is important when doing Pilates. Participants need to focus on the way their bodies move. They also need to be aware of how they are breathing.

Pilates is a favorite exercise of dancers and celebrities. Athletes often do Pilates to prevent or recover from injury. Pilates movements can be changed to match different fitness levels. This means almost anyone can do Pilates.

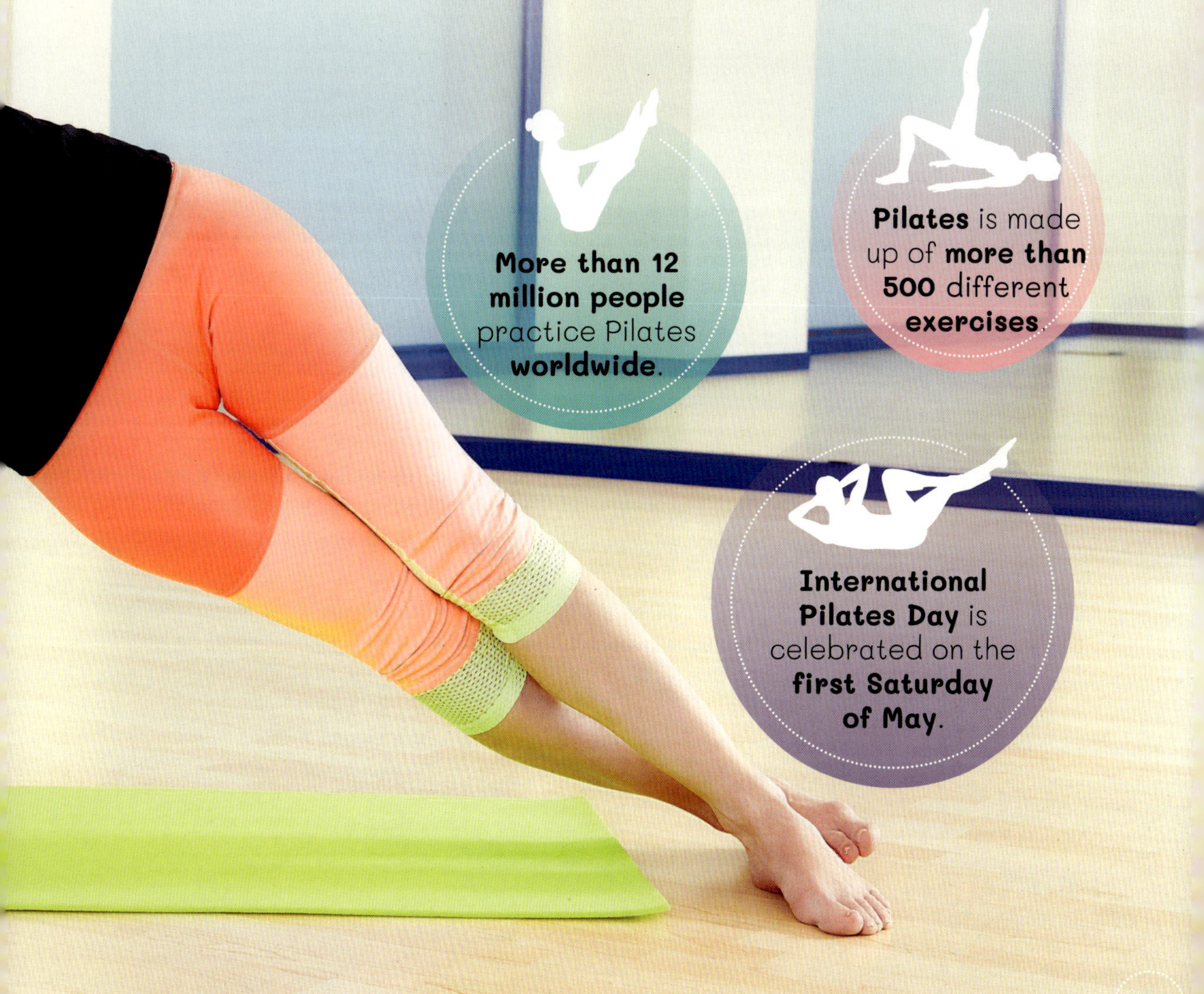

More than 12 million people practice Pilates **worldwide**.

Pilates is made up of **more than 500** different **exercises**.

International Pilates Day is celebrated on the **first Saturday of May**.

How It Started

German-born Joseph Pilates was often sick as a child. He suffered from asthma and other illnesses. Joseph fought to overcome his poor health. He turned to exercise to gain his strength back. Joseph was even able to become both a professional athlete and a circus performer.

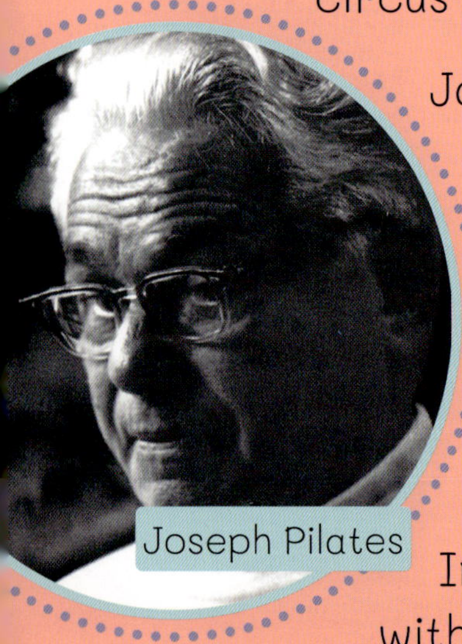

Joseph Pilates

Joseph wanted to help other people come back from illness and injury. During World War I, he developed exercises that wounded soldiers could do in their beds. After the war, Joseph continued to help people gain physical strength and stay fit.

In 1926, Joseph moved to New York City with his wife, Clara. They opened a fitness studio where they taught Joseph's unique form of exercise. They called it Contrology because it required participants to control their bodies, minds, and spirits. Over time, Contrology became known as Pilates.

The studio became well known. Members of New York's dance community took classes there to improve their muscle tone. As word spread about the benefits of Pilates, more people began practicing and teaching it. Today, more than 9 million people do Pilates on a regular basis in the United States alone.

Timeline

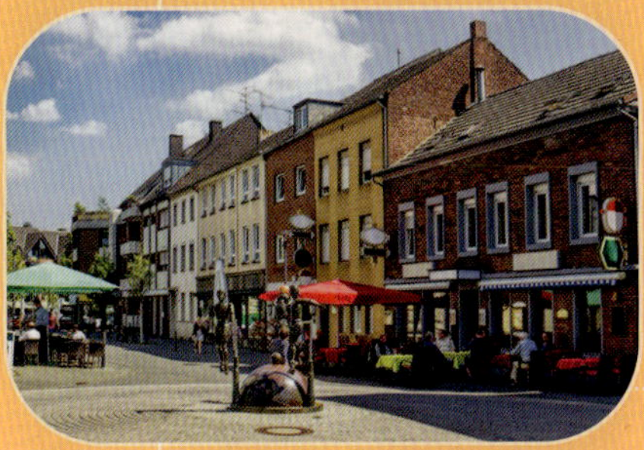

1883 Joseph Pilates is born in Mönchengladbach, Germany.

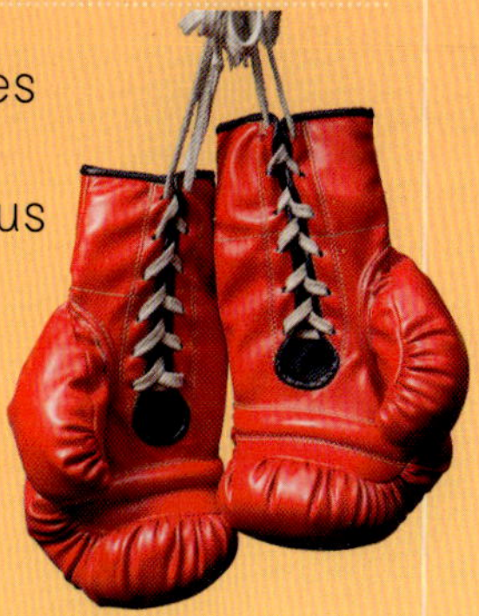

1912 Joseph lives in England and works as a circus performer, boxer, and self-defense instructor.

1926 Joseph and Clara move to New York City, where they open a fitness studio.

1945 Joseph publishes a book called *Return to Life Through Contrology*.

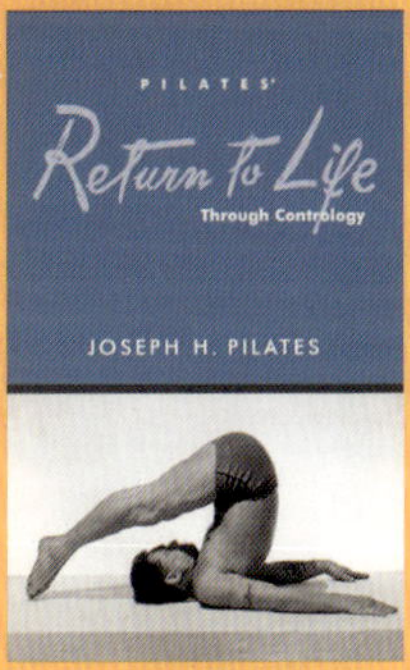

1967 Joseph dies at the age of 83.

2021 Apple adds Pilates workouts to its watch's fitness platform.

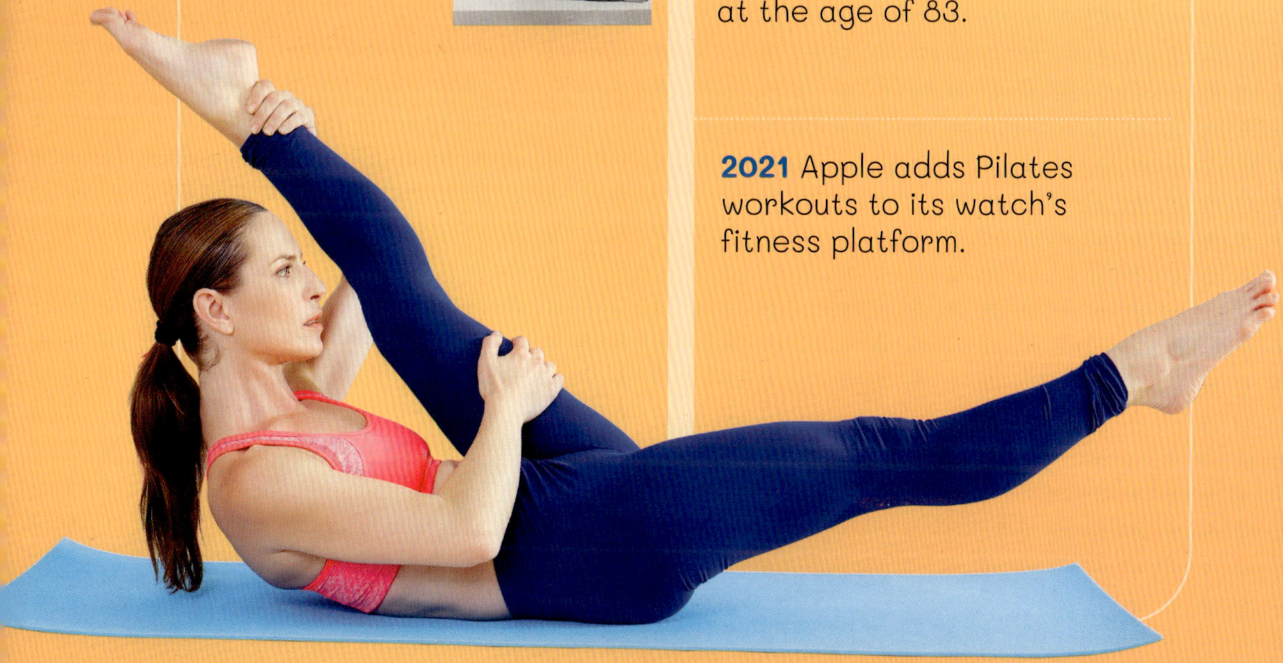

Ready for Pilates

Pilates can be done almost anywhere. However, studios are the best choice for those who want to use a range of equipment. People are encouraged to wear stretchy, form-fitting clothes to Pilates classes. They allow the body to move freely and stay covered. It is also a good idea to have a water bottle nearby. Staying **hydrated** is important during any exercise.

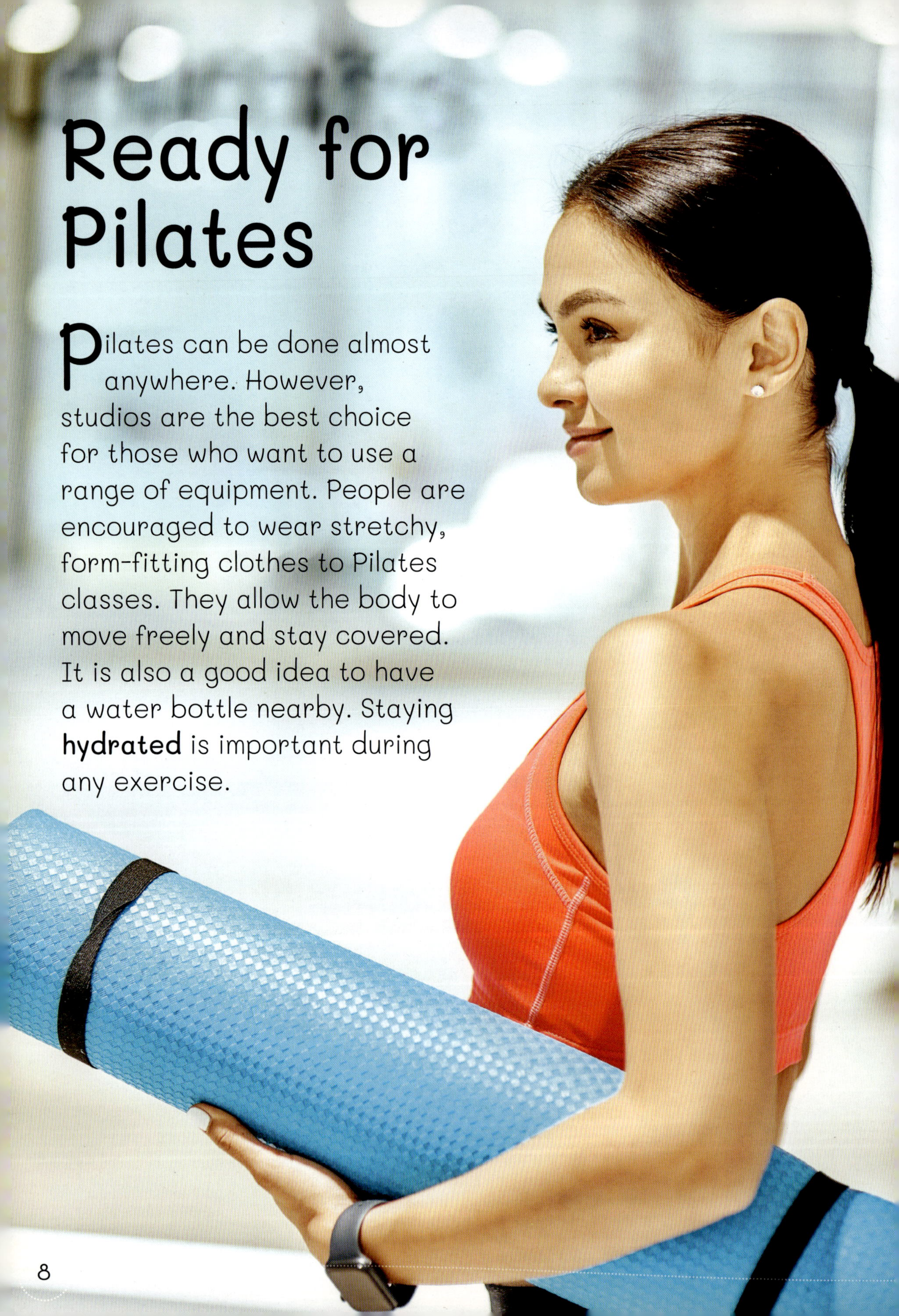

Equipment

Pilates exercises use **gravity** and a person's body weight to provide **resistance**. This is why many Pilates classes require only a mat. However, other equipment can also be added to a Pilates workout to help people through the exercises or provide more challenges.

Mat

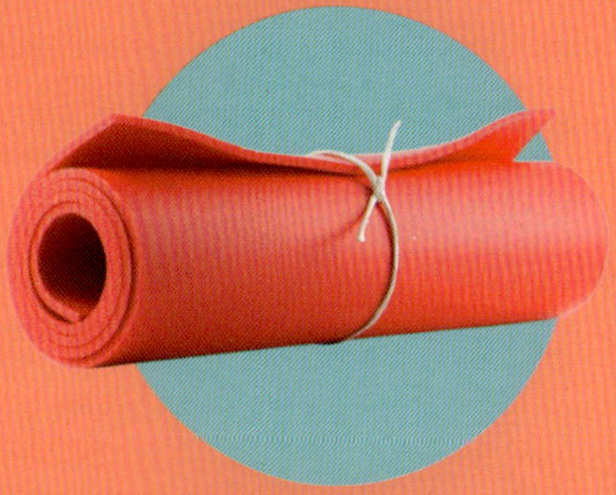

A mat is the most common item used in Pilates. Pilates mats tend to be thicker than those used in yoga. This provides cushioning and support for the body during floor movements.

Resistance Band

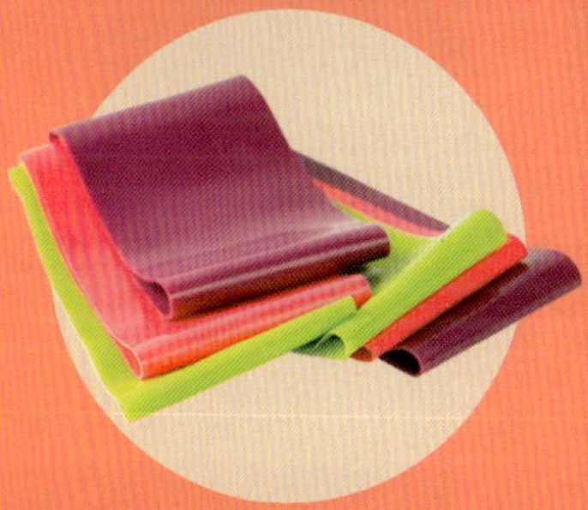

These stretchy plastic bands are used to strengthen and stretch the muscles. They add resistance to an exercise because the body must push against them to complete a movement. This can add a new level of challenge to a workout.

Stability Ball

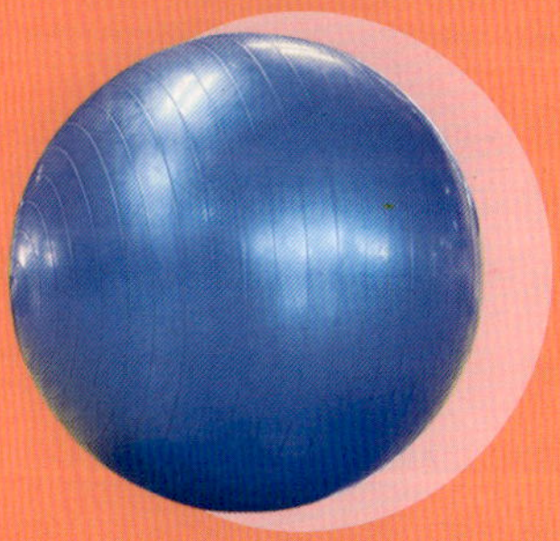

Introducing a stability ball to Pilates exercises can help people improve their balance and strengthen their core. By sitting or leaning over the ball, the body will try to stay stable. It will use a range of muscles to do this.

Reformer

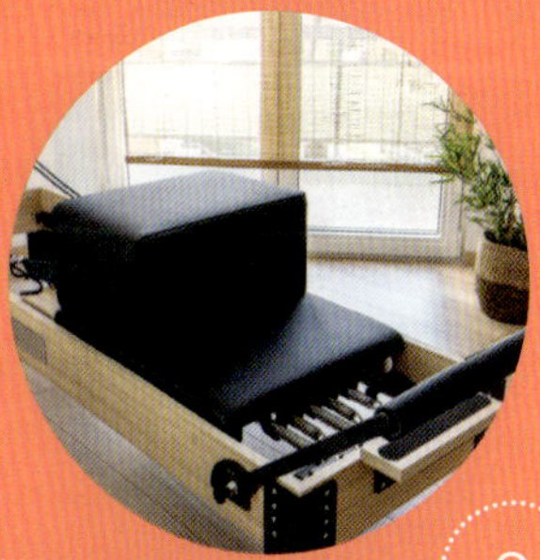

This piece of equipment is common in Pilates studios. It looks like a bed frame with a sliding platform. There are springs at one end that provide resistance during exercises. They move when ropes are pushed or pulled.

Getting Started

There are three main types of pilates workouts. Mat workouts involve floor exercises that require very little equipment. **Apparatus** workouts use reformers and other machines. Some classes use both mats and machines. No matter which type of workout is being done, all Pilates classes follow a similar format.

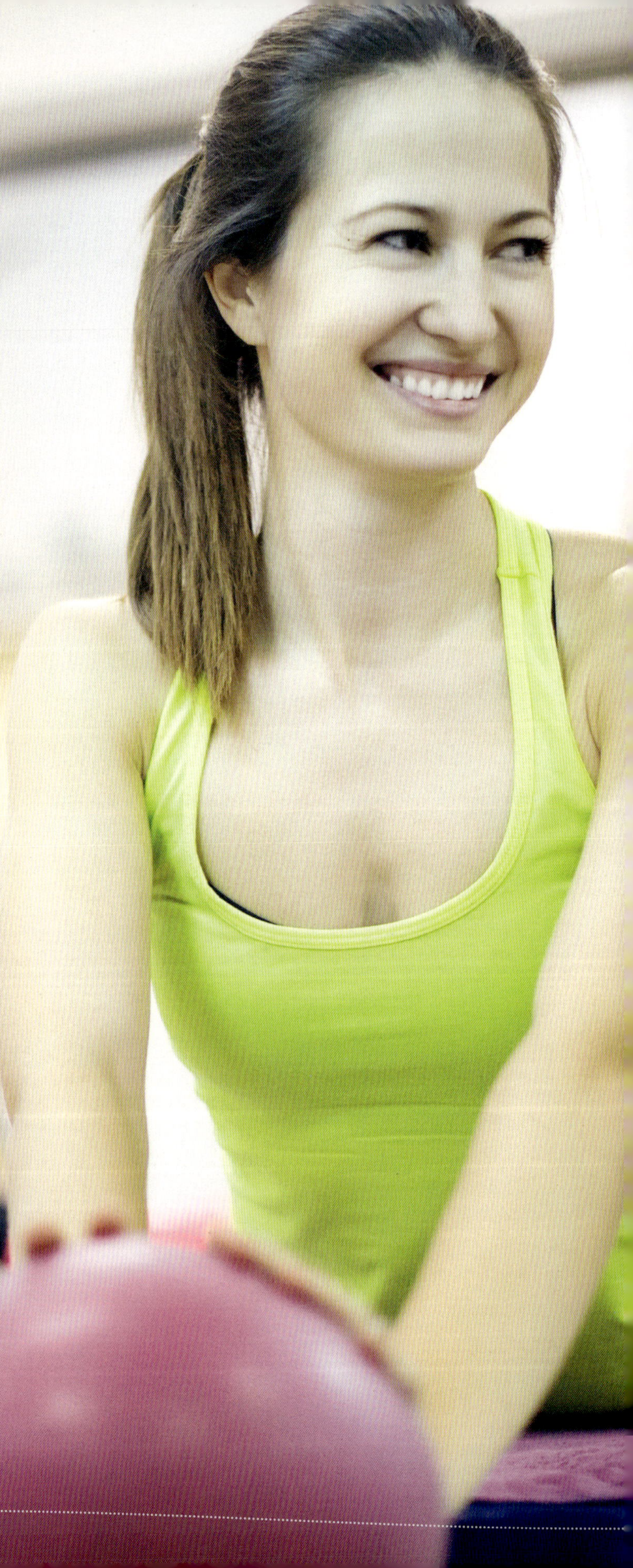

The beginning of a Pilates session typically starts with a warmup. The teacher will usually start by having students find their **neutral spine**. One way to do this is by lying flat on the back while pressing and releasing the lower spine into and out of the mat or platform. This exercise helps to ensure that the spine is **aligned** properly before any more exercises are done.

Once everyone has found their neutral spine, the class progresses to other moves. These may include head nods, shoulder rolls, foot circles, hip rotations, and arm openings. Each one of these moves helps prepare the body for the exercises done in class.

Throughout the warmup, the teacher will remind everyone to be mindful of their breathing. The warmup may even include some breathing exercises.

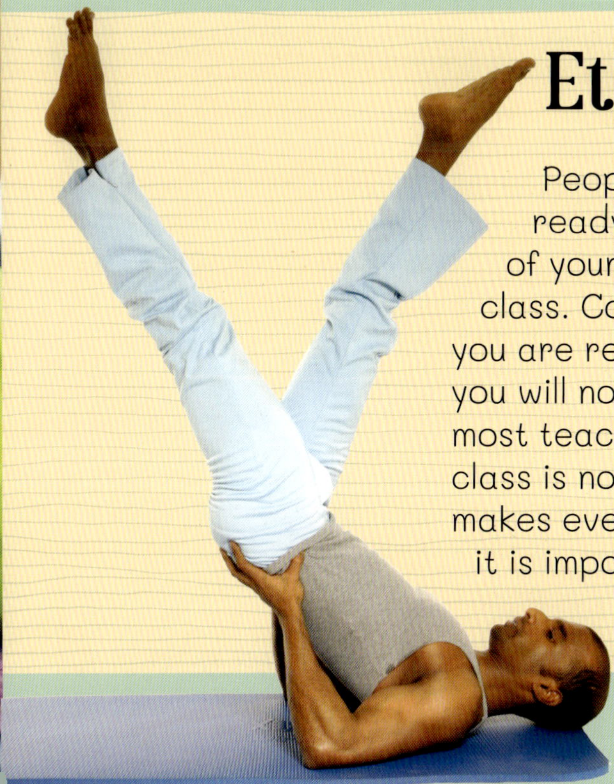

Etiquette

People should come to a Pilates class ready to focus and work. Be respectful of your teacher and the others in the class. Come a few minutes early so that you are ready when the class starts. This way, you will not distract your classmates. While most teachers encourage questions, a Pilates class is not a place to talk or visit. Chatter makes everyone lose their focus. This is why it is important to make sure that your phone is turned off during class as well.

Get Engaged

Joseph Pilates believed that all movement comes from the core, or "powerhouse." Most Pilates movements revolve around the core muscles for this reason. During class, Pilates teachers will often tell students to engage their core. This means they should tighten their core muscles so that they are ready for action. Having an engaged core will keep the spine stable and ensure that it does not become strained or injured.

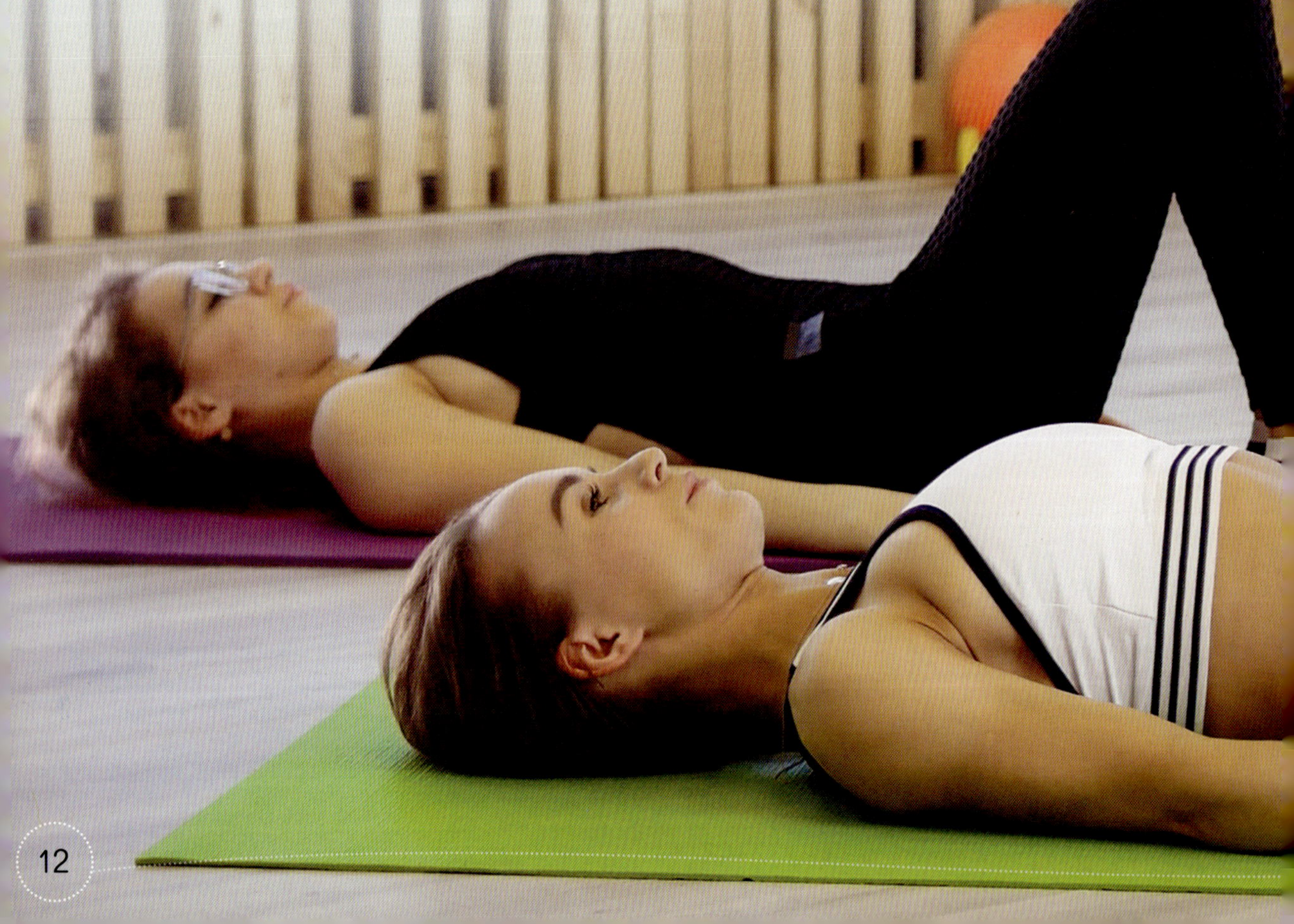

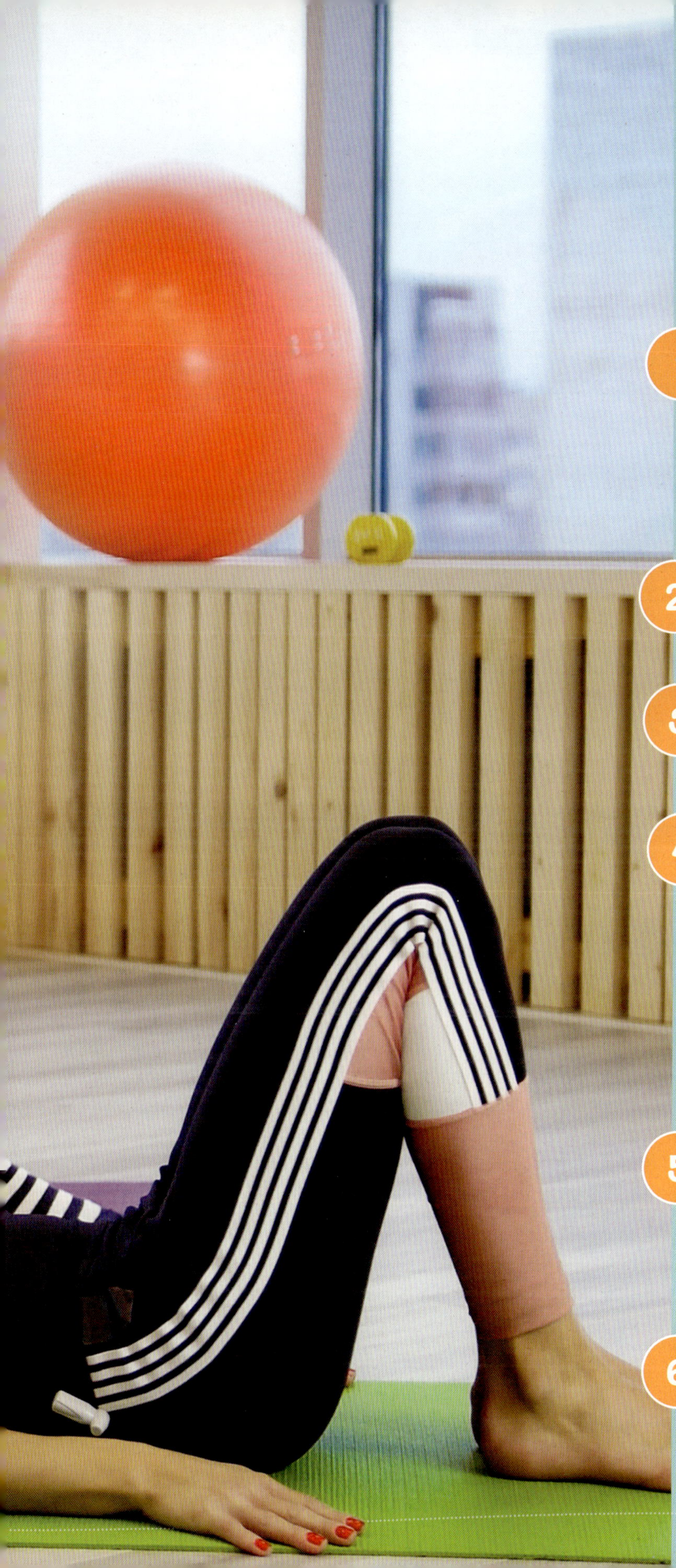

Try this exercise to engage your core muscles.

1. Lie with your back down on the floor and your knees slightly bent. Rest your arms flat along your body with the palms down.
2. Press your lower back into the floor.
3. Breathe in deeply and fill your belly with air.
4. Squeeze your stomach muscles to bring your belly button up toward your ribs and in toward your spine. Remember to keep your lower back on the floor.
5. Take three or four breaths, keeping your belly tight. Allow only your rib cage to move.
6. Relax your muscles and return to normal. Repeat this any time you want to engage your core.

In Control

During a Pilates class, a teacher guides students through a series of exercises. Most of these are done in sets of five or ten. They are often completed in a specific order. Each exercise must also follow the six core principles of Pilates.

1. **Centering** All movement should come from the center of the body.

2. **Concentration** Participants should bring their full attention to each move.

3. **Control** Every exercise should be done with deliberate and controlled movement.

4. **Precision** Participants must be aware of how each part of the body aligns with other parts.

5. **Breath** Air should be deeply pumped in and out of the body while exercising.

6. **Flow** Transitions between movements should be fluid and graceful.

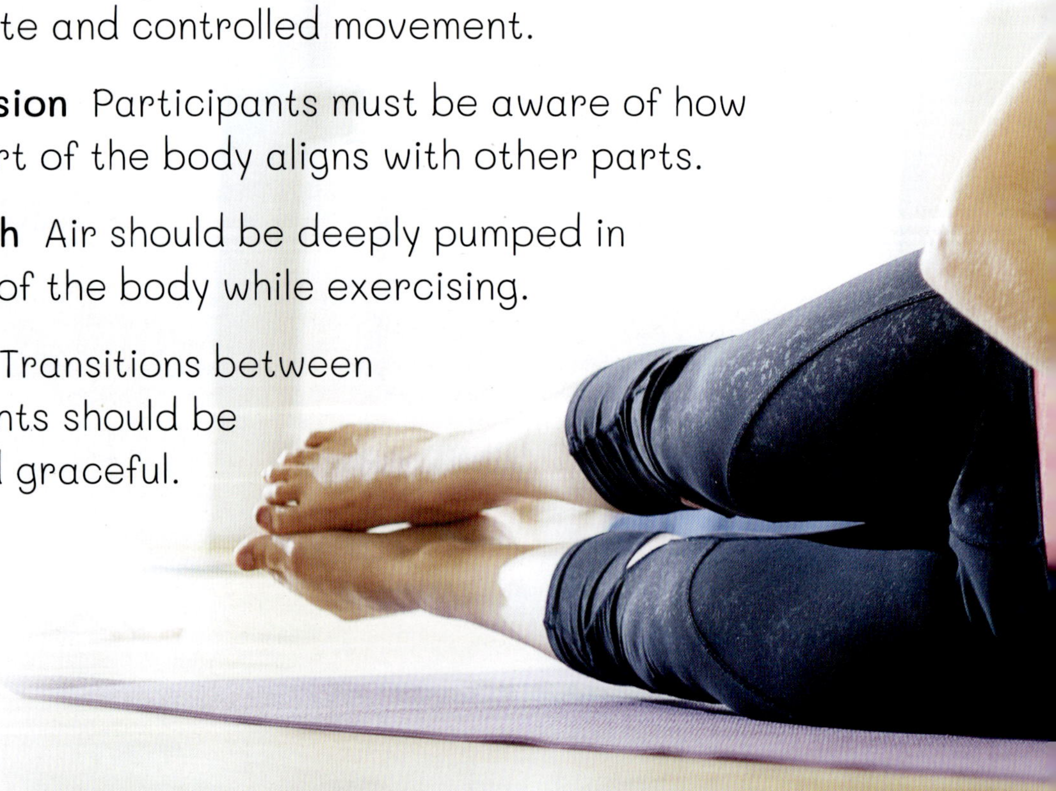

Pilates teachers typically move around during class. This allows them to check on everyone's body position and make sure people are exercising properly. It is common for Pilates teachers to correct people's alignment and movement using touch. A Pilates teacher will also tell students when to inhale and exhale during each exercise.

Pilates classes usually take 45 to 60 minutes. They can be held in silence or with quiet music. This allows students to focus on the exercises and the movement of their bodies.

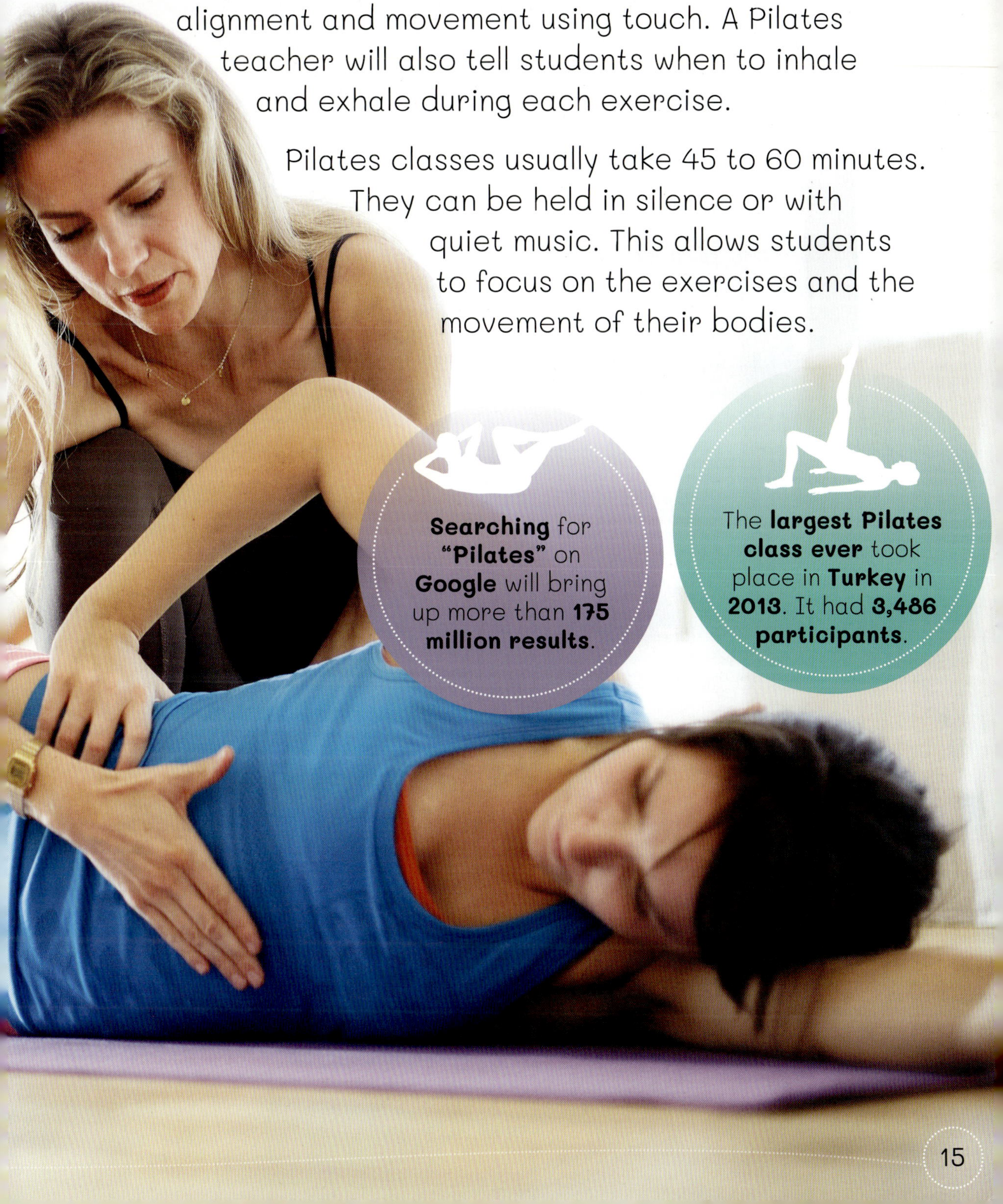

Searching for **"Pilates"** on **Google** will bring up more than **175 million results**.

The **largest Pilates class ever** took place in **Turkey** in **2013**. It had **3,486 participants**.

Pilates Moves

The Hundred, Swan, and Rolling Like a Ball are three of the most common exercises performed in mat classes. They are also popular moves for people new to Pilates. Taking Pilates classes is the best way to make sure correct **techniques** are being used. After that, mat exercises can be done at home.

The Hundred

The Hundred is named after the 100 beats made by the arms while the head, shoulders, and legs are lifted off the mat.

1. Lie on your back with your knees bent and feet on the floor.
2. Raise your legs so your knees are above your hips and your shins are **parallel** with the floor.
3. Inhale. Then, exhale and lift your head and shoulders off the ground, keeping your chin down toward your chest.
4. Inhale. Then, exhale and lift your arms a few inches from the floor, keeping them straight.
5. Hold this position and move your arms up and down while taking five short breaths in and five short breaths out.
6. Keep holding your legs, shoulders, and head up while you repeat the previous step 10 times.

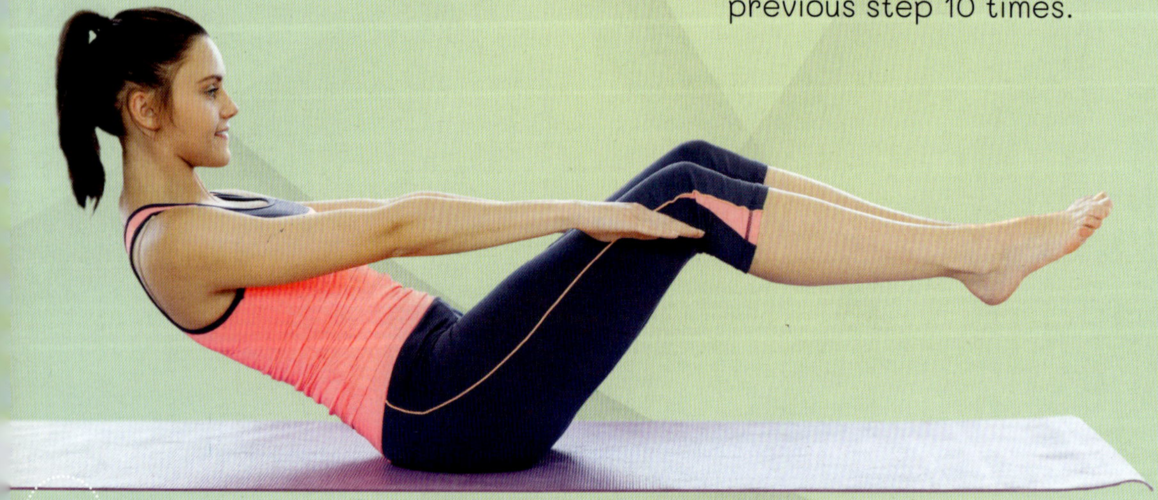

Swan

Swan works to strengthen hip, stomach, and arm muscles. It can also help to ease back pain.

1. Lie on your belly with your legs straight and your forehead touching the mat.
2. Bring your hands under your shoulders, keeping your bent elbows close to your body.
3. Lift your belly button away from the mat to engage your core.
4. Inhale and lengthen your spine as you lift your head and chest to form a slight arc.
5. Exhale and lower your forehead back to the mat.
6. Repeat Swan three to five times using an even, flowing breath.

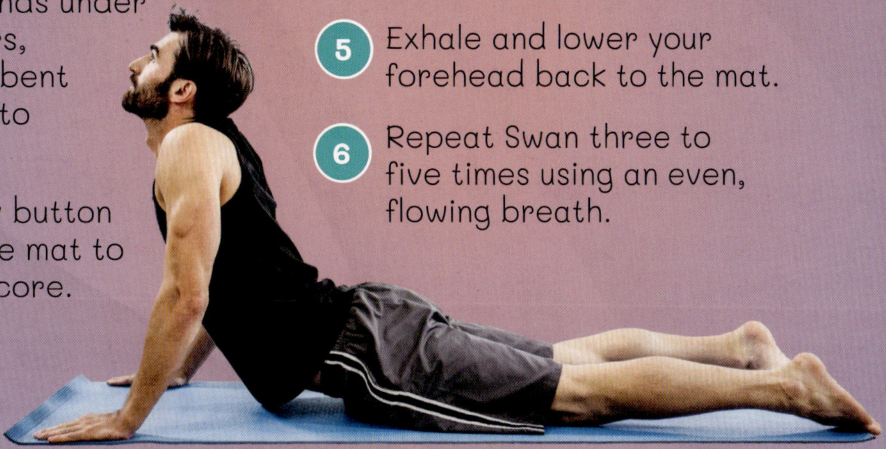

Rolling Like a Ball

This Pilates exercise provides a nice back massage. It requires the body to rock back and forth while rolled up in a ball.

1. Sit on your Pilates mat and clasp your hands over your shins, just above the ankle.
2. Drop your shoulders and engage your core. Tuck your chin so that you are looking down toward your belly button.
3. Lift your feet off the mat and balance yourself on your **sit bones**.
4. Inhale and roll back onto the shoulders.
5. Pause.
6. Exhale and use your core muscles to pull yourself back up.
7. Repeat this five to six times, keeping your back curved.

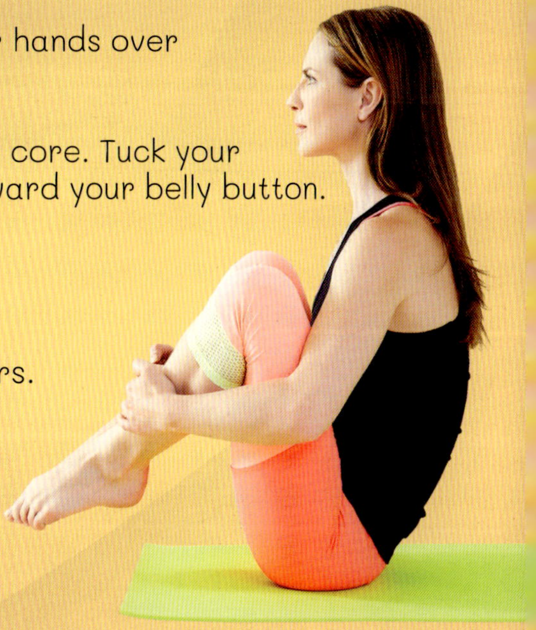

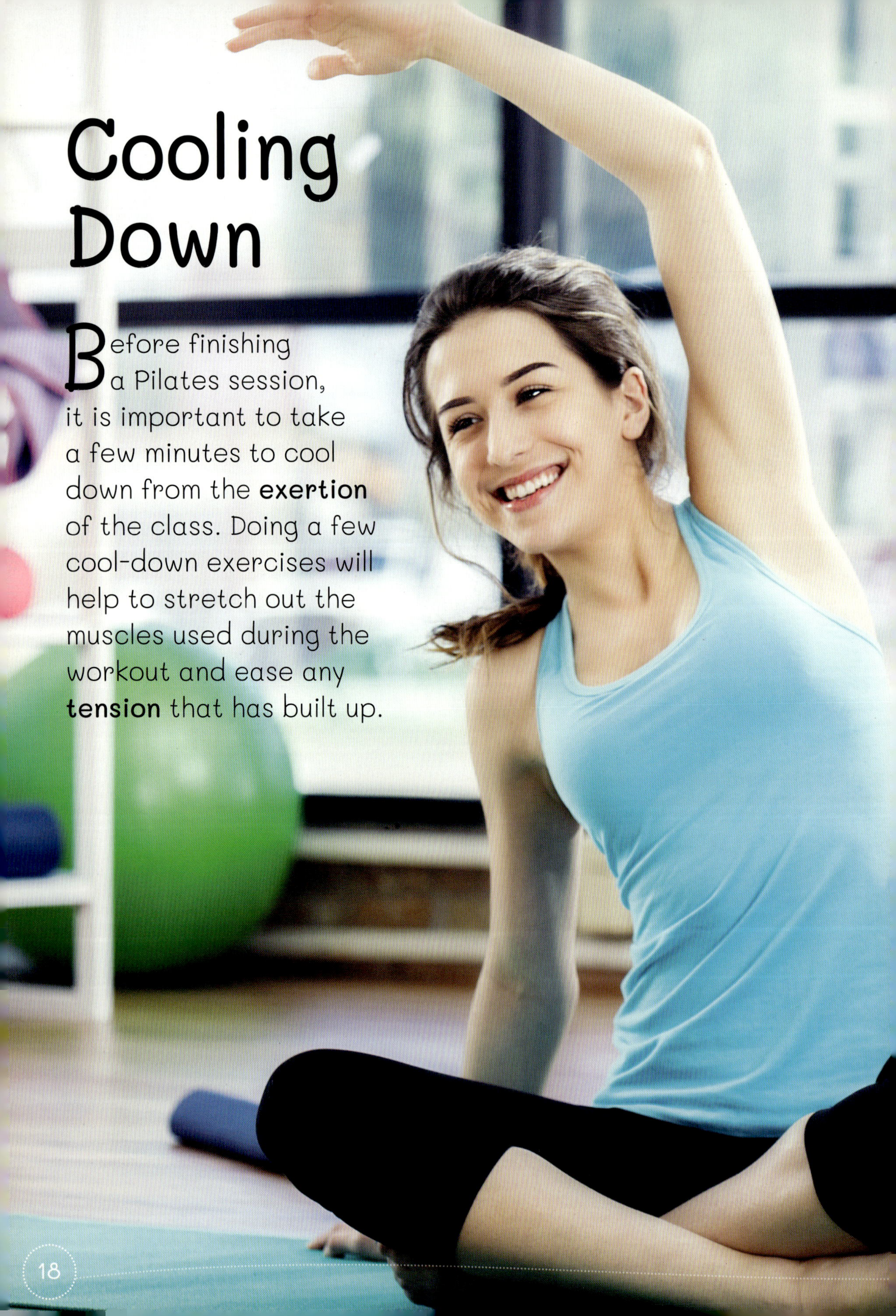

Cooling Down

Before finishing a Pilates session, it is important to take a few minutes to cool down from the **exertion** of the class. Doing a few cool-down exercises will help to stretch out the muscles used during the workout and ease any **tension** that has built up.

A Pilates teacher will usually take students through several cool-down exercises before ending a class. To stretch their necks, students may be asked to circle their heads in clockwise and counter-clockwise directions. They may stretch out their backs by sitting down and reaching for their toes. In all cases, cool-down exercises allow the body to gradually ease away from the intense activity it has just completed.

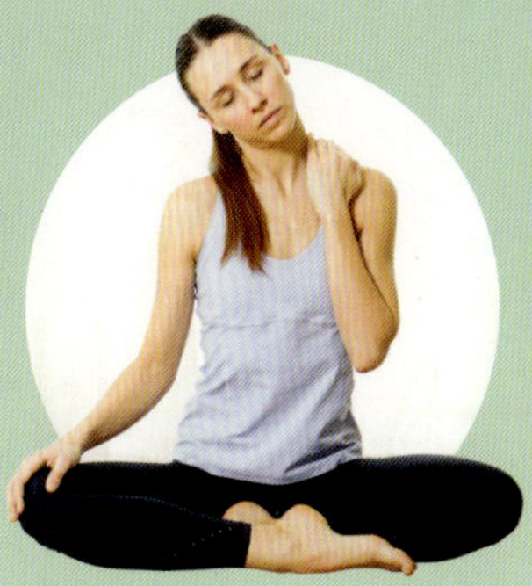

Even with a proper cool down, muscles are often sore after Pilates. This usually means they have been challenged and are working in new ways. As the body adjusts to the exercises and develops strength, this soreness will become less of a problem.

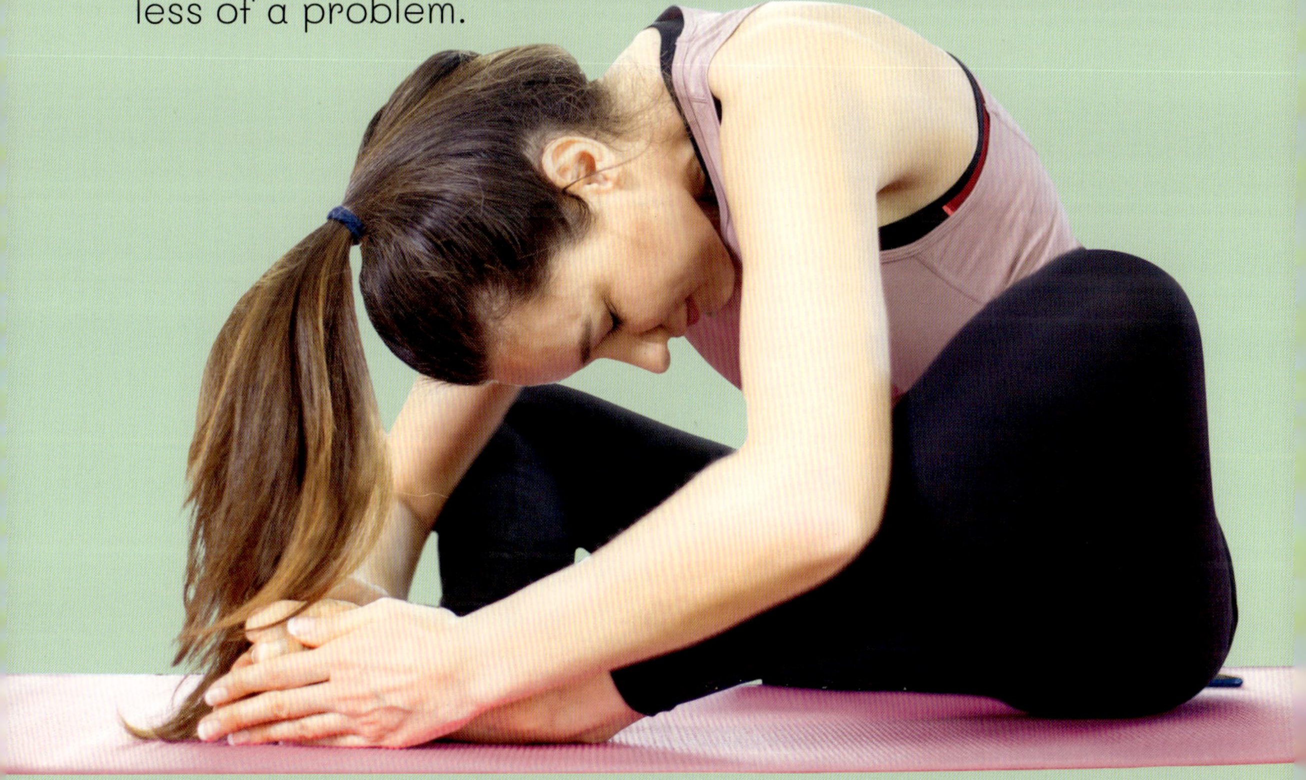

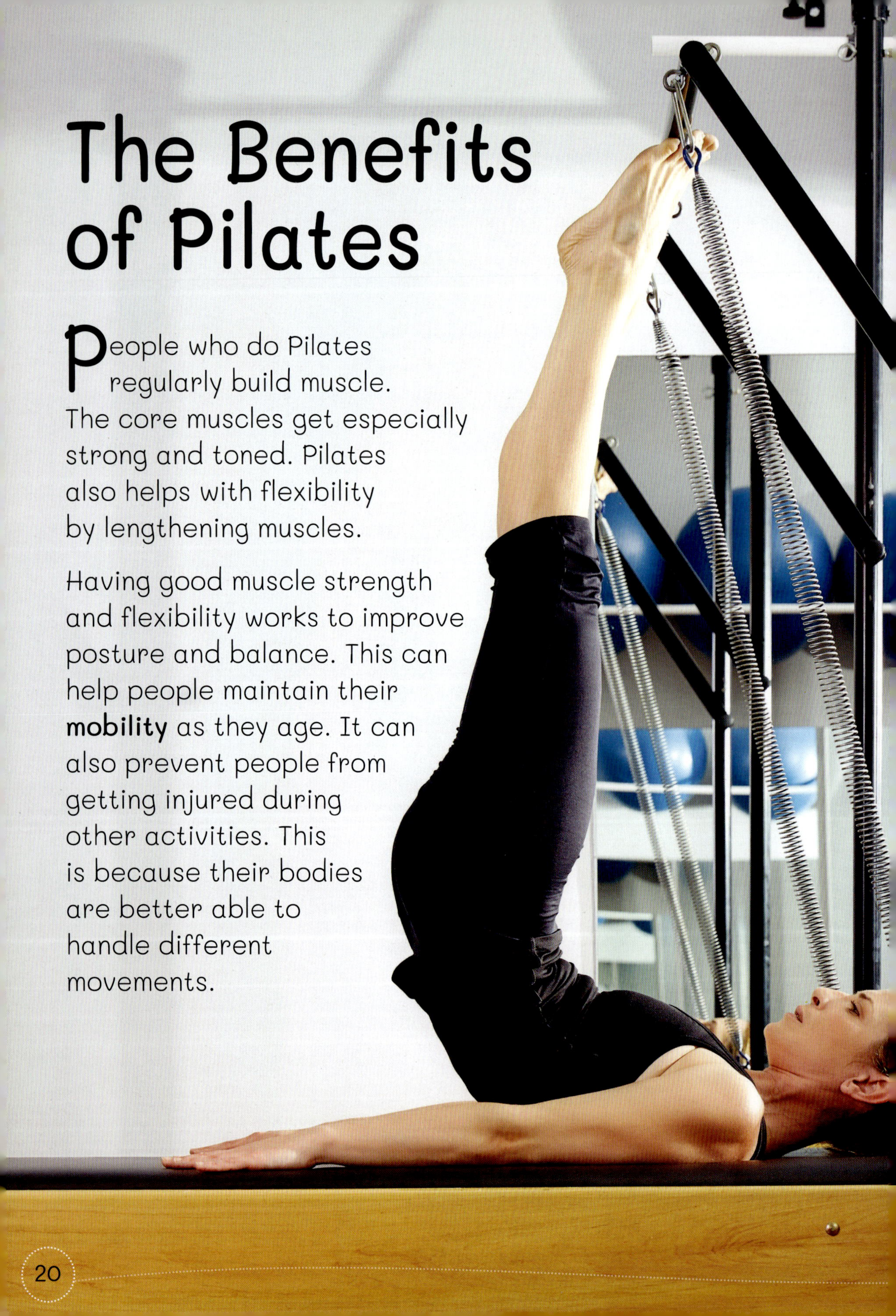

The Benefits of Pilates

People who do Pilates regularly build muscle. The core muscles get especially strong and toned. Pilates also helps with flexibility by lengthening muscles.

Having good muscle strength and flexibility works to improve posture and balance. This can help people maintain their **mobility** as they age. It can also prevent people from getting injured during other activities. This is because their bodies are better able to handle different movements.

When injuries do occur, Pilates can aid in recovery. Its low-impact format allows people to build up their strength without overly exerting themselves. Pilates can help people with back pain. This is because it targets the core muscles that support the back.

In addition to its physical benefits, Pilates is good for a person's mental health. The focus required to do Pilates can reduce **stress** levels and improve concentration. Pilates also promotes a strong mind-body connection. This encourages a sense of well-being.

Just **one hour** of **Pilates** will **burn calories** throughout the day.

More than 80 percent of the people taking **Pilates classes** are **women**.

When **Joseph Pilates** created **Contrology**, it had only **34 mat exercises**.

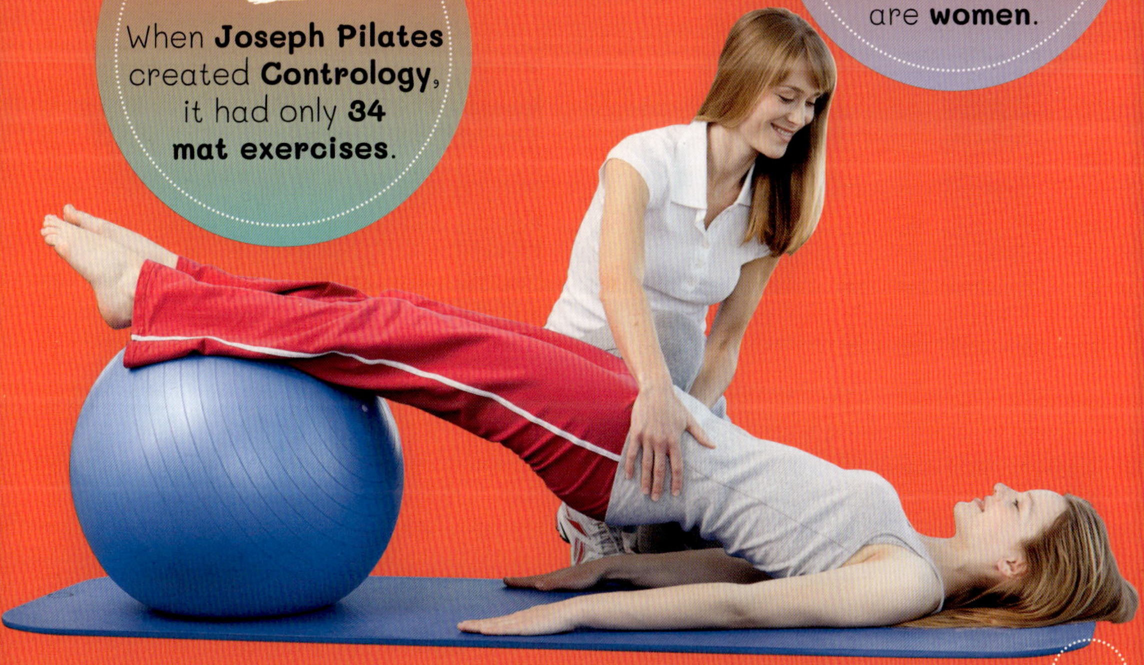

Pilates Quiz

1. What was Pilates first called?
2. How many people practice Pilates worldwide?
3. Who invented Pilates?
4. What do Pilates exercises use to provide resistance?
5. What is the most common type of equipment used in Pilates?
6. What are the three main types of Pilates workouts?
7. Around which muscles do Pilates exercises revolve?
8. What are the six core principles of Pilates?
9. How long is a typical Pilates class?
10. Which group makes up 80 percent of all people taking Pilates classes?

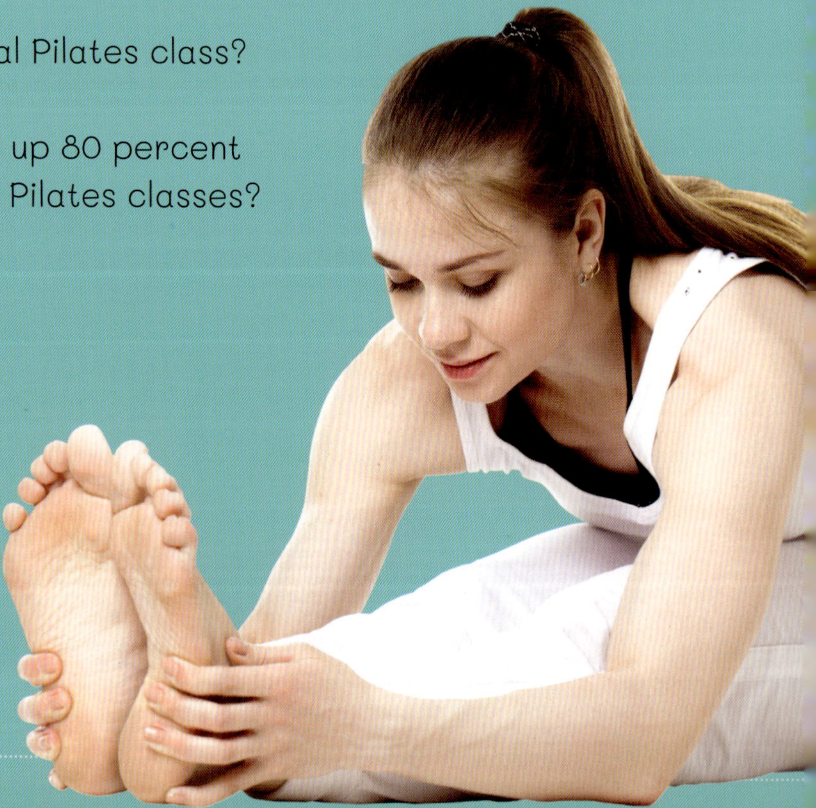

ANSWERS

1. Contrology **2.** More than 12 million **3.** Joseph Pilates **4.** Gravity and a person's body weight **5.** Pilates mat **6.** Mat, apparatus, and combination workouts **7.** Core muscles **8.** Centering, concentration, control, precision, breath, and flow **9.** 45 to 60 minutes **10.** Women

Key Words

aligned: in the correct position

apparatus: machines or tools that have a specific function

core muscles: the muscles in the torso, including those in the stomach and lower back

exertion: significant physical or mental effort

flexibility: the ability to bend easily

gravity: the force that pulls objects to the center of Earth

hydrated: having enough water

mobility: the ability to move freely

neutral spine: the position in which the spine maintains its natural curves

parallel: being the same distance apart at all points

posture: the way people hold their bodies when sitting, standing, or walking

precision: accuracy and exactness

resistance: one force that works against the motion of another

sit bones: the bones at the bottom of the pelvis that make contact with a surface when a person is sitting down

stress: a state of mental or emotional strain

techniques: special ways of carrying out an activity

tension: the state of being stretched or strained

Index

Get the best of both worlds.

AV2 bridges the gap between print and digital.

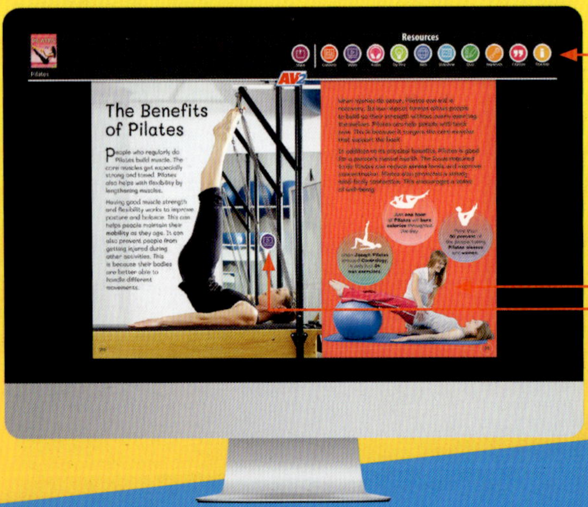

The expandable resources toolbar enables quick access to content including **videos**, **audio**, **activities**, **weblinks**, **slideshows**, **quizzes**, and **key words**.

Animated videos make static images come alive.

Resource icons on each page help readers to further **explore key concepts**.

Published by Lightbox Learning Inc.
276 5th Avenue, Suite 704 #917
New York, NY 10001
Website: www.openlightbox.com

Library of Congress Cataloging-in-Publication Data

Name: Ridge, Yolanda, 1973- author.
Title: Pilates / Yolanda Ridge.
Description: New York, NY : AV2, 2023. | Series: Wellness : mind body motion | Includes index. | Audience: Grades 2-3
Identifiers: LCCN 2021033651 (print) | LCCN 2021033652 (ebook) | ISBN 9781791142599 (library binding) | ISBN 9781791142605 (paperback) | ISBN 9781791142612
Subjects: LCSH: Pilates method--Juvenile literature. | Mindfulness (Psychology)--Juvenile literature.
Classification: LCC RA781.4 .R54 2022 (print) | LCC RA781.4 (ebook) | DDC 613.7/192--dc23
LC record available at https://lccn.loc.gov/2021033651
LC ebook record available at https://lccn.loc.gov/2021033652

Printed in Guangzhou, China
1 2 3 4 5 6 7 8 9 0 25 24 23 22 21

122021
101121

Project Coordinator: Heather Kissock
Designer: Terry Paulhus

Photo Credits
Every reasonable effort has been made to trace ownership and to obtain permission to reprint copyright material. The publisher would be pleased to have any errors or omissions brought to its attention so that they may be corrected in subsequent printings. The publisher acknowledges Getty Images, Alamy, and Shutterstock as its primary photo suppliers for this title.